KNOWLEDGE GUIDE TO
PAGET'S DISEASE

Essential Manual To Symptoms, Diagnosis, Treatment Options, and Long-term Management

DR. AARON BRANUM

Copyright © 2024 BY DR. AARON BRANUM

All rights reserved. Except for brief quotations embodied in critical reviews and certain other noncommercial uses permitted by copyright law, no part of this publication may be reproduced, distributed, or transmitted in any form or by any means, Including photocopying, recording, or other electronic or mechanical methods, without the prior written permission of the publisher.

Disclaimer:

The data in this book, is solely meant to be informative and instructional.

This book is not intended to replace expert medical advice, diagnosis, or care. No medical, health, or other professional services are offered by the author, publisher, or any affiliated parties

Individual outcomes may differ in the practice of these therapies, which entail a variety of approaches and methodologies.

A one-on-one session with a trained or certified healthcare professional is still preferable. It is best to consult a trained healthcare provider before making any decisions regarding your health.

The author of this book is not affiliated with any specific website, product, or organization related to any of these therapies.

All reasonable measures have been taken by the author and publisher to guarantee the authenticity and dependability of the material contained in this book

Contents

CHAPTER ONE 17

  THE PATHOPHYSIOLOGY OF THE DISEASE PAGET 17

    Process Of Bone Remodeling 17

    Osteoblasts And Osteoclasts' Roles 18

    Unusual Growth Of Bones In Paget's 18

    Mechanisms Of The Spread Of Illness 19

    Effect On The Bone Structure 20

CHAPTER TWO 23

  PAGET'S DISEASE TYPES 23

    Paget's Monostotic 23

    Polyostotic Paget's 25

    Deformable Osteitis 27

    Variations And Presentations In Clinical Practice 28

    Uncommon Types And Subtypes 30

CHAPTER THREE 33

  DIAGNOSIS AND ASSESSMENT 33

    Clinical Evaluation 33

    Imaging Studies (CT, MRI, And X-Rays) ... 34

Laboratory Tests (Bone Turnover Markers, Alkaline Phosphatase)...........................35

Procedures For Biopsies 36

Distinctive Diagnosis 36

CHAPTER FOUR 39

MODALITIES OF TREATMENT 39

Drugs..39

Procedures Surgical...............................41

Rehabilitation And Physical Therapy.........42

Techniques For Pain Management............43

Changes In Lifestyle 44

CHAPTER FIVE 45

COPING WITH THE DISEASE OF PAGET 45

Support Networks And Coping Mechanisms 45

Consistent Monitoring Is Essential 47

Guidelines For Exercise And Nutrition.......49

Handling Soreness And Unease 52

Sustaining Life Quality 54

CHAPTER SIX...59

OBSTACLES AND PROGNOSIS...................59

Breaks And Deformities Of The Bone 59

   Loss Of Hearing And Neurological Issues .. 60

   Cardiovascular Symptoms 61

   Possibility Of Adjacent Conditions
   (Osteosarcoma) 62

   Prognostic Factors And Long-Term Outlook
   63

CHAPTER SEVEN 65

   RESEARCH AND PROGRAMS 65

   Trends In Current Research 65

   New Therapeutic Strategies 66

   Studies In Genetics And Molecular Biology 68

   Clinical Trial Involvement And Patient
   Engagement 69

   Prospects For The Future Of Paget's Disease
   Treatment 71

CHAPTER EIGHT 73

   COMMONLY ASKED QUESTIONS OR FAQS .. 73

   Is Paget's Bone Disease Genetic? 73

   Exists A Cure For Paget's Disease? 74

What Adjustments To Your Lifestyle Can Help Manage Paget's Disease? 75

Steer Clear Of High-Impact Activities: 76

Exist Any Other Options For Treating Paget's Disease? 77

How Frequently Should I Contact My Healthcare Provider Again? 78

CONCERNING THIS BOOK

The "Knowledge Guide to Paget's Disease of Bone" is an essential tool for anyone looking for a thorough grasp of this complicated ailment, regardless of whether they are a medical professional or not. This book navigates through its different facets with clarity and detail, explaining everything from the nuances of Paget's Disease to its diagnosis, treatment, and the difficulties of living with it.

Fundamentally, the book explores the substance of Paget's Disease, dissecting its definition and offering a thorough synopsis. By means of thorough investigation, it clarifies the causes, risk factors, symptoms, and diagnostic procedures, equipping readers with the necessary knowledge to identify and promptly treat the illness.

The investigation of the pathophysiology of Paget's Disease, which sheds light on the bone remodeling process, the function of osteoclasts and osteoblasts, and the causes driving aberrant bone formation, is fundamental to the book's effectiveness. Studying the sorts of Paget's Disease, including monostotic and polyostotic variants, deepens readers' comprehension of its clinical variances and presentations, even going into rare forms and subtypes.

Readers are guided through clinical assessment, imaging investigations, laboratory testing, biopsy procedures, and differential diagnosis, enabling a comprehensive and accurate diagnosis, with the help of insights into diagnosis and evaluation. In addition, the book carefully describes a range of therapeutic modalities, including physical therapy, rehabilitation, and lifestyle changes in addition to drugs and surgery, encouraging a comprehensive approach to illness management.

As it delves into the world of living with Paget's Disease, the book offers priceless advice on coping mechanisms, networks of support, and the significance of routine monitoring. It covers recommendations for diet and exercise, methods for managing pain, and the importance of preserving quality of life despite the difficulties the illness presents.

Furthermore, the book navigates the landscape of consequences and prognosis, offering information on fractures, bone deformities, hearing loss, neurological issues, cardiac symptoms, and the possibility of secondary illnesses such as osteosarcoma. It advances the conversation by exploring new frontiers in genetics, and molecular biology, developing therapeutic options, and current research trends, providing an outlook on the management of Paget's Disease.

The book answers commonly asked questions, debunking myths, bringing clarification, and giving comfort to those who are facing uncertainty. With its compelling story and thorough analysis, "Knowledge Guide to Paget's Disease of Bone" proves to be an invaluable resource, providing understanding, strength, and hope for anyone dealing with this complex illness.

Defining and summarizing

A chronic disorder known as Paget's disease of the bone results in aberrant remodeling of the bone, which weakens and malforms the bone.

It can affect one or more bodily bones and usually affects older persons. The illness can cause a range of symptoms, from minor to severe, and usually advances slowly over time.

The natural cycle of bone regeneration and repair is disturbed with Paget's disease, which results in the production of weaker, larger, and malformed bones.

Complications like fractures, arthritis, and nerve compression may arise from this. Although the precise etiology of Paget's disease remains unclear, genetic predispositions and viral infections have been linked to its progression.

Reasons and Danger Elements

Although the exact etiology of Paget's disease is still unknown, a number of factors may be involved in its onset. Given that the illness typically runs in families, genetics is a major factor. Furthermore, there may be an infectious component to Paget's disease because some viral infections, including the paramyxovirus, have been connected to it.

Given that Paget's disease primarily affects people over 50, age is another important risk factor. Men are more likely than women to be impacted, and European Americans are more likely to be afflicted than members of other ethnic groups.

Environmental variables that can raise the chance of getting Paget's disease include exposure to specific chemicals or poisons.

Signs and Symptoms

Many symptoms may appear in people with Paget's disease of the bone, while some people may go for extended periods of time without experiencing any symptoms.

Bone abnormalities, joint stiffness, and bone pain are common symptoms. Engaging in physical exercise or bearing weight might exacerbate pain and suffering.

Complications from Paget's illness might occasionally include nerve compression, hearing loss, and fractures. Bone abnormalities can also happen, such as bending of the legs or a curved spine.

Furthermore, because of the increased blood flow to the affected location, the bones may feel warmer to the touch.

Diagnostic Examinations

A combination of the patient's medical history, physical examination, and imaging testing is usually used to diagnose Paget's disease.

Alkaline phosphatase is a blood marker that can be used to assess bone turnover.

A common sign of Paget's illness is elevated alkaline phosphatase levels.

Imaging studies can be used to see abnormalities in the bones and determine the extent of bone involvement.

Examples of these procedures are MRIs, X-rays, and bone scans. X-rays can show distinctive alterations including larger, thicker bones with a "mosaic" pattern of bone remodeling.

Whereas MRI scans offer fine-grained images of soft tissue and bone structures, bone scans can identify regions with elevated bone activity.

Difficulties

Many consequences, from minor to severe, can result from Paget's disease of the bone. Bone fractures are among the most frequent side effects, and they can be brought on by weakening or brittle bones. Fractures, especially in weight-bearing bones like the hips or spine, can result in discomfort, incapacity, and decreased mobility.

Osteoarthritis is another consequence of Paget's disease that can occur in joints with malformations in the bone.

Nerve compression can happen when swollen bones press against nearby nerves, causing symptoms like tingling, numbness, or weakness in the affected area.

 Although it is not very frequent, Paget's illness can occasionally lead to osteosarcoma or bone cancer.

CHAPTER ONE

THE PATHOPHYSIOLOGY OF THE DISEASE PAGET

Process Of Bone Remodeling

It is essential to comprehend the normal bone remodeling process in order to comprehend Paget's disease of the bone.

Bone rejuvenation is an ongoing process that involves a dynamic equilibrium between the creation and resorption of bone.

Osteoclasts and osteoblasts are the two main cell types that are in charge of this process. Whereas osteoblasts create new bone in its place, osteoclasts are in charge of dissolving outdated or damaged bone tissue. Bone integrity and strength are ensured by this delicate equilibrium.

Osteoblasts And Osteoclasts' Roles

Originating from the same stem cells as macrophages, osteoclasts are the main cells in charge of bone resorption.

They release calcium and other minerals into the bloodstream by secreting acids and enzymes that break down the mineralized bone matrix.

On the other hand, the development of bones is the responsibility of osteoblasts. Collagen and other proteins that make up the organic matrix of bone are produced and secreted by them. This matrix then turns mineralized, forming new bone tissue.

Unusual Growth Of Bones In Paget's

This equilibrium between osteoblast-mediated bone production and osteoclast-mediated bone resorption is upset in Paget's disease.

Excessive osteoclast activity results in a rise in bone resorption.

Following this phase of hyperactive bone resorption, osteoblast activity increases in response, leading to an overabundance of disorderly bone production.

Characteristic traits like bigger or malformed bones result from the new bone that grows, which is frequently structurally aberrant, larger, and weaker than normal bone.

Mechanisms Of The Spread Of Illness

Although the precise cause of Paget's disease is still unknown, a number of factors are thought to play a role in its development. Due to the disease's tendency to run in families, genetic factors are involved.

Furthermore, among vulnerable individuals, viral infections, specifically caused by the paramyxovirus, have been linked to the onset of the condition. But not everyone infected by these viruses goes on to suffer Paget's disease, indicating a major role in genetic predisposition.

Effect On The Bone Structure

Depending on which bones are impacted, the aberrant bone development associated with Paget's disease might result in different consequences.

Increased bone density can cause discomfort, deformity, and an increased risk of fractures in weight-bearing bones like the spine or pelvis.

Unusual growth in the skull bones can cause neurological issues like migraines, hearing loss, and abnormalities in vision because they compress surrounding structures.

Additionally, since the heart has to work harder to pump blood via these engorged veins, the increased blood flow to afflicted bones may put certain people at risk for heart failure. Comprehending these anatomical alterations is essential to effectively addressing Paget's disease consequences.

CHAPTER TWO

PAGET'S DISEASE TYPES

Paget's Monostotic

A type of Paget's disease of the bone known as monostotic Paget's disease affects only one damaged bone.

Compared to polyostotic Paget's disease, this form is less prevalent, but it is still important to recognize its characteristics in order to make a correct diagnosis and provide the right therapy. While monostotic Paget can affect any bone in the body, it usually affects the pelvis, femur, and lumbar spine, which are all weight-bearing bones.

An imbalance between bone production and resorption results from aberrant remodeling of the afflicted bone in monostotic Paget's disease. The bone may become weaker, larger, and misshapen as a result of this. When radiographic imaging is done for other purposes and the disease is only discovered through it, patients may have localized discomfort, tenderness, or even periods of no symptoms.

MRIs, bone scans, and X-rays are examples of diagnostic imaging that is essential for diagnosing monostotic Paget's disease.

Bone expansion, cortical thickening, and regions of radiolucency and sclerosis are frequently observed radiographic findings. The goal of treatment is to manage symptoms.

Pain management techniques, bisphosphonates, and, in certain situations, orthopedic treatments to address structural issues may be used to halt the process of bone remodeling.

Polyostotic Paget's

A more common form of Paget's disease where numerous bones are damaged is called polyostotic disease. In contrast to the monostotic variant, polyostotic Paget's disease can affect multiple bone sites at once. Bones such as the pelvis, spine, skull, and long bones of the legs are frequently afflicted.

Similar pathophysiological alterations to those observed in monostotic Paget's disease are present in this variant of the disease, resulting in aberrant bone remodeling and structurally disorganized and larger bones in each affected bone.

Due to changed biomechanics, patients may develop broader symptoms such as skeletal abnormalities, secondary arthritis in neighboring joints, increased fracture risk, and bone discomfort.

More serious systemic problems, such as elevated cardiac output as a result of the overactive bone tissue's metabolic needs, might result from polyostotic Paget's disease.

A combination of clinical assessment, blood testing (high alkaline phosphatase levels), and imaging studies are usually used to make the diagnosis.

Treatment plans frequently involve pain medication, physical therapy, bisphosphonates, calcitonin, and, if necessary, surgical treatments to fix fractures or repair abnormalities.

Deformable Osteitis

Paget's disease of the bone is also known as osteitis deformans, referring to the distinctive abnormalities that develop in the afflicted bones.

This phrase emphasizes the disease's inflammatory component, which involves the diseased bones' ongoing remodeling and inflammation.

Osteitis deformans is characterized by the formation of thicker but structurally weaker bones.

This process is the outcome of an excessive bone tissue breakdown that is followed by a disordered creation of new bone. Affected bones may become malformed, resulting in physical abnormalities like bowed legs, swollen skulls, or curvy spines.

Osteitis deformans patients can exhibit a variety of symptoms, such as joint pain from involvement in nearby joints, bone discomfort, and problems like a hearing loss if the skull is affected.

Because the disease is chronic, long-term management plans are necessary, with the main goals of treatment being to reduce symptoms and regulate the process of bone remodeling.

This frequently entails the use of calcitonin and bisphosphonates in addition to supporting therapies including physical rehabilitation and pain relief methods.

Variations And Presentations In Clinical Practice

Because Paget's disease of the bone can show a wide variety of clinical symptoms, diagnosis and management of this disorder can be challenging. The bones affected and the severity of the disease can have a substantial impact on the symptoms.

Localized bone pain is a common clinical manifestation. It can be continuous or sporadic, and it can get worse when you move. Additionally, skeletal abnormalities such as leg bending or larger skulls may be noticed by patients. Because many patients may be asymptomatic in the early stages, there are situations in which the disease is unintentionally found through imaging done for unrelated purposes.

Additional clinical variables include neurological problems, such as spinal stenosis or radiculopathy resulting from nerve compression syndromes affecting the vertebrae.

Because of the compression of cranial nerves, patients with skull involvement may endure headaches, hearing loss, or even visual issues.

Paget's disease can proceed slowly or rapidly and aggressively, depending on the clinical course.

This variety calls for a customized approach to diagnosis and therapy, with ongoing clinical evaluations, blood tests, and imaging studies to monitor the course of the illness and the effectiveness of the chosen course of action.

Uncommon Types And Subtypes

Although monostotic or polyostotic variants account for the bulk of instances of Paget's disease, there are unusual forms and subtypes that pose particular difficulties.

Among these is juvenile Paget's disease, an extremely uncommon hereditary variant that manifests in childhood or adolescence and is distinguished by severe malformations and extensive bone involvement.

Paget's disease of the spine is another uncommon subgroup in which there are serious structural and neurological problems due to vertebral involvement.

Serious back pain, spinal instability, and compression of the spinal cord or nerve roots may arise from this, calling for intricate treatment plans that can involve surgery.

Paget's sarcoma is an extremely uncommon but dangerous consequence in which the afflicted bone undergoes a malignant change. Because of its aggressive nature, this subtype needs to be treated with chemotherapy, radiation therapy, and surgery as soon as possible.

It is essential to identify these uncommon forms and subtypes in order to treat affected patients appropriately and enhance their prognoses.

It entails a high degree of suspicion, a comprehensive clinical assessment, and a multidisciplinary approach to care.

CHAPTER THREE

DIAGNOSIS AND ASSESSMENT

Clinical Evaluation

Clinical examination is an essential component in the diagnosis of Paget's disease of the bone. It entails a thorough assessment of the symptoms and medical background of the patient.

Physicians will ask if the patient has ever had any fractures, abnormalities, or pain in their bones.

They might also search for symptoms like warmth or soreness over the afflicted bones, as these could be indicators of active inflammation.

A physical examination is also performed to evaluate mobility and any obvious anomalies, such as malformations or enlarged bones.

Imaging Studies (CT, MRI, And X-Rays)

In order to diagnose and assess Paget's disease of the bone, imaging investigations are crucial. Since X-rays are easily accessible and may identify common abnormalities in the bone, like enlargement, thickness, and sclerosis, they are frequently utilized as the first imaging modality.

More comprehensive pictures can be obtained with MRI and CT scans, which are especially helpful for determining the extent of bone involvement, identifying potential problems including nerve or spinal cord compression, and directing surgical planning as needed.

Laboratory Tests (Bone Turnover Markers, Alkaline Phosphatase)

In order to diagnose Paget's disease of the bone and track the disease's progression, laboratory testing is a useful adjuvant. Measuring serum levels of alkaline phosphatase, an enzyme produced by osteoblasts (cells involved in bone production), is one of the important assays.

Patients with Paget's disease usually have elevated levels of alkaline phosphatase, which is indicative of accelerated bone turnover.

Moreover, bone resorption and formation rates can be assessed using bone turnover markers including serum collagen type I cross-linked C-telopeptide (CTX) and serum N-terminal propeptide of type I collagen (PINP), which help with disease monitoring and therapy response assessment.

Procedures For Biopsies

Biopsies may be done in some situations to confirm the diagnosis or rule out other bone ailments, even though they are rarely required for the diagnosis of Paget's disease of the bone. A biopsy is the process of taking a little sample of bone tissue, either during surgery or a minimally invasive treatment like a needle biopsy. A pathologist next looks through the collected tissue under a microscope to check for abnormalities that are typical of Paget's disease, such as increased vascularity, disorganized bone structure, or multinucleated large cells.

Distinctive Diagnosis

In order to differentiate Paget's disease of the bone from other illnesses that may exhibit comparable symptoms or radiographic findings, differential diagnosis is crucial. Osteoporosis, osteoarthritis, bone metastases, and other bone dysplasias are known to resemble Paget's disease.

The pattern of bone involvement, the existence of distinctive radiographic characteristics, and the outcomes of laboratory testing are important differentiators.

To provide an accurate diagnosis and create a suitable treatment plan, healthcare professionals from several professions, such as radiologists, orthopedic surgeons, and rheumatologists, may need to work together.

CHAPTER FOUR

MODALITIES OF TREATMENT

Drugs

Bisphosphonates

The most often given drugs for Paget's disease of the bones are bisphosphonates. These medications function by preventing osteoclasts—the cells that resorb bone—from doing their job. Bisphosphonates aid in normalizing the bone remodeling process by lowering bone turnover, which promotes the creation of stronger and more structurally sound bones. Risedronate, zoledronic acid, and alendronate are examples of commonly used bisphosphonates. These drugs can be injected intravenously or taken orally, though intravenous administration is frequently chosen due to its strength and longer duration of action. In order to rapidly get the condition under control, treatment typically begins with a larger dose and is then continued at maintenance levels in order to prevent recurrence.

Calcitonin

Another treatment for Paget's disease is the hormone calcitonin, which is generated by the thyroid gland. This drug prevents osteoclasts from resorbing bone and helps control the body's calcium levels.

For people who cannot handle bisphosphonates, calcitonin is an option, however less frequently used than bisphosphonates due to its lower potency. Usually, nasal spray or injection is used to give it. In order to evaluate the efficacy of the treatment and make any appropriate modifications, routine monitoring is required.

Procedures Surgical

Surgical intervention may be required if Paget's disease results in consequences such as severe bone deformities, fractures, or osteoarthritis. Orthopedic surgery can replace arthritis-damaged joints, fix fractures, and rectify abnormalities.

For instance, if the hip joint is seriously damaged, a total hip replacement may be necessary to provide significant pain relief and increased mobility.

If the spinal cord or nerves are compressed, spinal surgery can be necessary. These are intricate treatments that need to be carefully planned and carried out by skilled surgeons.

Rehab following surgery is essential to get the optimum result.

Rehabilitation And Physical Therapy

An essential part of treating Paget's disease of the bones is physical therapy. A physical therapist can create a customized exercise program that will help strengthen muscles, increase mobility, and improve overall function. The basic goals of exercises are to increase muscle strength, flexibility, and balance—all of which are essential for preserving independence and avoiding falls.

Because water-based activities are low-impact and less taxing on the bones and joints, aquatic therapy can be very advantageous. In order to reduce stress on injured bones, physical therapists often instruct their patients on good posture and body mechanics.

Techniques For Pain Management

For people with Paget's disease to live better lives, effective pain management is crucial. The initial line of treatment is frequently pain medications such as acetaminophen or nonsteroidal anti-inflammatory medicines (NSAIDs).

Doctors may recommend stronger drugs, including opioids or muscle relaxants, for patients experiencing more severe pain. Apart from pharmaceutical interventions, non-pharmacological methods such as massage, acupuncture, and heat and cold therapy can also be helpful. Patients may find it easier to manage their chronic pain and lessen its effects on everyday life with the use of cognitive-behavioral therapy (CBT) and other psychological interventions.

Changes In Lifestyle

People with Paget's disease can greatly benefit from making specific lifestyle adjustments. Bone health depends on eating a balanced diet high in calcium and vitamin D. Weight-bearing activities like walking and lifting weights enhance general fitness and help build bones. It's crucial to abstain from smoking and binge drinking because these behaviors might harm your bones. It's critical to follow up with medical professionals on a regular basis to track the disease's course and modify treatment as needed. Mobility and safety can be improved by using assistive equipment like walkers or canes, especially for people who have severe bone abnormalities or balance problems.

CHAPTER FIVE

COPING WITH THE DISEASE OF PAGET

Support Networks And Coping Mechanisms

There are many obstacles to overcome when dealing with Paget's Disease, both psychologically and physically.

Support networks and coping mechanisms are essential for successfully handling these difficulties. In order to effectively cope, it's critical to keep lines of communication open with loved ones, friends, and healthcare professionals.

Through this contact, people can voice their worries, exchange experiences, and ask for help when they need it.

In addition, support groups can be very helpful for those with Paget's Disease.

Members of these organizations are able to relate to each other's experiences, which fosters a sense of understanding and camaraderie. Knowing that one is not traveling alone can be consoling and reassuring when stories, pointers, and counsel are exchanged inside these communities.

People must learn internal coping strategies in addition to receiving outside assistance. To help manage stress and anxiety, this may involve engaging in mindfulness practices like meditation or deep breathing exercises. Discovering enjoyable and soothing pursuits, like hobbies or time spent in nature, can also enhance general well-being.

Moreover, retaining an optimistic perspective can significantly impact an individual's ability to manage the difficulties associated with having Paget's Disease.

Keeping an optimistic and resilient mindset can be achieved by concentrating on the positive elements of life, making reasonable goals, and acknowledging and appreciating all of life's accomplishments, no matter how tiny.

Consistent Monitoring Is Essential

To properly manage Paget's Disease and avoid complications, routine monitoring is crucial. This entails routine check-ups, symptom monitoring, and therapy efficacy assessment at medical facilities.

Regular monitoring allows medical professionals to evaluate bone health, monitor the disease's course, and modify treatment regimens as necessary.

Numerous procedures and evaluations, such as blood tests to gauge bone turnover marker levels, imaging examinations like X-rays or bone scans to appraise bone integrity and structure, and clinical assessments to gauge symptoms and general health, may be part of the monitoring process.

Early intervention can help prevent problems like fractures, deformities, or nerve compression.

Early detection of changes in bone health or disease development allows for rapid intervention. Furthermore, routine monitoring gives medical professionals a chance to answer any queries or worries patients may have regarding their condition or course of treatment.

Maintaining optimal bone health and overall well-being is contingent upon proactive engagement in routine monitoring for those diagnosed with Paget's Disease.

People can actively manage their illness and lessen the burden of the disease on their lives by being informed, being honest with healthcare practitioners, and following suggested monitoring regimens.

Guidelines For Exercise And Nutrition

In order to manage Paget's Disease and promote general bone health, diet and exercise are essential. Maintaining strong and healthy bones requires a diet rich in key nutrients, including calcium and vitamin D.

A balanced diet is crucial for this. Foods high in calcium include dairy products, almonds, leafy greens, and fortified cereals; foods high in vitamin D include fatty fish, egg yolks, and fortified foods.

Regular exercise is essential for promoting bone strength and density, in addition to a healthy diet.

Exercises that include lifting weights, such as dancing, running, weightlifting, or walking, can promote bone formation and lower the chance of fractures.

Strengthening your muscles and increasing bone density can also be achieved with resistance training, such as lifting weights or resistance bands.

But before beginning any new fitness program, people with Paget's Disease must use caution and speak with their healthcare practitioners. Some activities might need to be avoided or modified in order to prevent harm or worsening of symptoms.

Personalized suggestions based on each patient's unique health condition and disease severity can be given by healthcare professionals.

In addition, it's critical to maintain a healthy body weight to lessen the load on the joints and bones.

A healthy weight can be attained and maintained with the aid of a balanced diet and frequent exercise, both of which can improve bone health and well-being in general.

Individuals diagnosed with Paget's Disease can improve their general quality of life, manage their symptoms, and maintain their bone health by adhering to individualized dietary and activity regimens.

Handling Soreness And Unease

One of the most prevalent signs of Paget's disease is pain, which can have a serious negative effect on quality of life.

A comprehensive strategy that takes into account the psychological as well as the physical components of pain is necessary for effective pain management.

Prescription drugs may be used to treat Paget's Disease-related pain and inflammation. For mild to moderate pain, nonsteroidal anti-inflammatory drugs (NSAIDs) like ibuprofen or naproxen may be used; for severe pain, a doctor may prescribe harsher pharmaceuticals like opioids.

To reduce hazards and adverse effects, it's crucial to use these drugs sparingly and under the supervision of medical professionals.

Various complementary therapies and lifestyle modifications can assist manage pain and discomfort in addition to pharmaceuticals. Physical therapy methods that relieve muscle tension and increase flexibility include massage, heat or cold therapy, and mild stretching exercises.

Acupuncture, chiropractic adjustments, and methods of relaxation like aromatherapy or guided imagery can also aid in pain relief and relaxation.

In order to effectively manage the pain and discomfort brought on by Paget's disease, emotional support is just as crucial. Support groups, counseling, and mindfulness-based techniques can assist people in managing the psychological effects of chronic pain and creating plans for keeping a positive mindset.

In addition, sustaining a healthy lifestyle that includes enough sleep, frequent exercise, and a good diet can help reduce pain and promote general well-being. People with Paget's Disease can enhance their quality of life and reclaim control over their health by managing their pain holistically and from a variety of perspectives.

Sustaining Life Quality

Keeping up one's quality of life is the main objective for those with Paget's Disease. Notwithstanding the difficulties the illness presents, there are a number of tactics and treatments that can support people in maintaining their general well-being and carrying on with their favorite hobbies.

Optimizing symptom management with a mix of medicinal interventions, lifestyle changes, and supportive therapies is essential to preserving quality of life.

This could involve taking drugs to reduce inflammation and pain, getting physical therapy to increase range of motion and function, and using assistive technology to help with everyday tasks.

Individuals with Paget's Disease must focus on holistic well-being and self-care in addition to symptom treatment.

This could be doing fun activities that encourage social interaction and relaxation, practicing stress-reduction methods like yoga or meditation, and asking for help from friends, family, and medical professionals.

For those who have Paget's Disease, maintaining a sense of meaning and purpose in life can also improve overall quality of life.

This could be establishing objectives, pursuing interests or hobbies, volunteering, or taking part in fulfilling and meaningful relationships and activities.

Furthermore, making educated decisions about one's health and available treatments can be facilitated by maintaining empowerment and knowledge about one's situation.

People can keep a sense of control and autonomy over their lives by actively taking part in their care and speaking out for their needs.

All things considered, preserving the quality of life in the face of Paget's Disease necessitates an all-encompassing, multidisciplinary strategy that takes into account social, emotional, and physical components of well-being.

People can improve their general quality of life and manage Paget's Disease by combining medical treatments, self-care routines, and supportive interventions.

CHAPTER SIX

OBSTACLES AND PROGNOSIS

Breaks And Deformities Of The Bone

Bones weakened and expanded by Paget's disease of the bone are more prone to fractures and abnormalities.

Because of the aberrant bone remodeling process, bones become more brittle and are not structurally sound. The pelvis, the spine, and the long bones of the arms and legs are common places for fractures.

These fractures can be especially crippling, resulting in decreased mobility and persistent pain. The illness can result in severe bone abnormalities like bent legs, enlarged skulls, or curved spines in addition to fractures.

In addition to affecting outward appearance, these deformities can also influence function and increase the risk of further issues, such as arthritis, because of changes in joint biomechanics.

Loss Of Hearing And Neurological Issues

Hearing loss is one of the more concerning effects of Paget's illness. This happens when the disease affects the skull's bones, specifically the temporal bone.

The hearing-related nerves may be compressed by the aberrant bone growth, or the ear's tissues may be affected. Consequently, partial or total hearing loss may occur in patients with Paget's illness.

Additionally, if the condition affects the skull or spine, neurological problems may result. Symptoms including discomfort, tingling, numbness, and weakening in the muscles can result from compression of the spinal cord or nerves. In extreme circumstances, it may lead to balance and coordination issues, which can seriously lower the quality of life.

Cardiovascular Symptoms

The cardiovascular system may be affected by Paget's disease. The heart may be under additional stress due to the increased blood flow to regions where bone remodeling is occurring.

Because of the enlarged vascular network inside the damaged bones, the heart must work harder to pump blood through this condition, also known as high-output cardiac failure.

This heart condition can cause exhaustion, breathing difficulties, and ankle and leg edema.

Despite being a relatively uncommon consequence, it is significant and needs to be treated by a physician in order to manage the symptoms and stop further heart problems.

Possibility Of Adjacent Conditions (Osteosarcoma)

Osteosarcoma, a kind of bone cancer, is the most serious secondary ailment that individuals with Paget's disease are more likely to acquire. This complication is uncommon, but because of its aggressive nature and dismal prognosis, it warrants serious attention.

Osteosarcoma symptoms might include fractures, observable swelling, and increasing bone pain.

Osteosarcoma diagnosis and management might be complicated by Paget's disease, although early discovery and treatment are essential for better outcomes. For those with severe or extensive Paget's disease, routine imaging studies and monitoring are advised to identify any early indications of malignant change.

Prognostic Factors And Long-Term Outlook

The prognosis for people with Paget's disease of the bones varies greatly and is dependent on a number of factors, such as the severity and extent of the disease, the particular bones afflicted, and the existence of comorbidities. Many patients with the condition have a milder version and are able to effectively control their symptoms with medication and lifestyle changes.

On the other hand, patients who have more severe consequences or a more widespread disease may have a more difficult prognosis.

The age of diagnosis, the efficacy of treatment, and the general health of the patient are prognostic factors that impact the long-term outlook.

For those with Paget's disease to have a better prognosis and quality of life, early identification and treatment are essential.

Effective illness management necessitates regular follow-up with healthcare providers, adherence to treatment plans, and monitoring for consequences.

CHAPTER SEVEN

RESEARCH AND PROGRAMS

Trends In Current Research

Considerable progress has been made in the last few years in the diagnosis and treatment of Paget's Disease of Bone (PDB). The growing emphasis on the disease's genetic foundations is one significant trend. Utilizing cutting-edge genomic tools, researchers are able to find genetic markers and mutations connected to PDB.

By identifying the inherited components of the illness, this genetic research hopes to shed light on why some people are predisposed to acquire PDB.

The emphasis on early diagnosis and action is another trend. Scientists are trying to identify

PDB in its early stages using advanced imaging methods and markers of bone turnover. Effective disease management and the avoidance of serious consequences depend on early identification.

In an effort to provide all-encompassing preventative methods, research is also looking into how lifestyle and environmental variables contribute to the development and progression of PDB.

New Therapeutic Strategies

PDB therapeutic research is developing quickly, and novel approaches to treatment are imminent.

The cornerstone of PDB treatment, bisphosphonates, is being improved for increased effectiveness and decreased side effects. In an effort to improve patient outcomes, researchers are looking into the possibilities of novel bisphosphonate formulations and alternative dosage schedules.

Innovative treatment drugs are being investigated in addition to bisphosphonates. Clinical trials indicate potential for monoclonal antibodies that target bone resorption mechanisms, such as denosumab. These biological medications offer a focused strategy that may help individuals who don't react well to conventional therapies.

PDB research is exploring an interesting new area: gene therapy. Researchers are looking into ways to fix genetic alterations at the cellular level in an effort to find a longer-lasting cure for the illness. Another cutting-edge strategy being investigated is stem cell therapy, which has the ability to rebuild healthy bone tissue and return to normal bone function.

Studies In Genetics And Molecular Biology

Studies in molecular biology and genetics have been essential to expanding our knowledge of PDB. Numerous genes, including SQSTM1, have been connected to the illness by researchers.

The distinctive bone defects observed in PDB are caused by mutations in these genes that interfere with normal bone remodeling mechanisms.

Scientists are learning more about the disease's underlying biological pathways by examining these genetic alterations. This information is essential for creating focused treatments that can alter or stop the illness process in its tracks. In order to better understand the intricate biology of PDB, researchers are also looking into the function of signaling networks and molecular interactions in bone cells.

Studies in molecular biology are also concentrating on finding biomarkers that can help with PDB monitoring and early diagnosis. These biomarkers may offer a non-invasive way to monitor the course of a disease and the effectiveness of a treatment plan, enhancing patient care and results.

Clinical Trial Involvement And Patient Engagement

The foundation of medical advancements in PDB is clinical trials. Testing the efficacy and safety of novel therapies and treatment modalities requires these trials.

Enrolling in clinical trials provides patients with access to novel medications that are not yet commercially available, which may enhance their quality of life.

PDB sufferers are being actively sought after by researchers for a range of scientific trials that address various facets of the illness, from innovative diagnostic methods to fresh pharmacological treatments.

Patient involvement is essential because it yields the data required to support innovative treatment development and commercialization.

Patient advocacy organizations and educational initiatives are essential for promoting trial participation.

The advancement of PDB research depends on these organizations' ability to maintain a consistent flow of participants by educating the public about the advantages and significance of clinical trials.

Prospects For The Future Of Paget's Disease Treatment

PDB management is expected to become increasingly accurate and tailored in the future. Approaches to personalized treatment are being made possible by developments in molecular biology and genetic research.

Treatments may be customized in the future based on a patient's genetic profile, increasing efficacy and reducing side effects.

Another interesting approach is the incorporation of digital health technologies. Real-time monitoring of bone health and disease progression could be made possible by wearable technology and mobile health applications, allowing for more proactive and responsive PDB treatment.

It is anticipated that diverse teams will collaborate more in order to tackle the challenges of PDB.

This cooperative strategy will probably hasten the creation of novel treatments and deepen our knowledge of the illness.

PDB management appears to have a bright future overall, as new research and technology developments are expected to change the way that patients are diagnosed, treated, and cared for.

CHAPTER EIGHT

COMMONLY ASKED QUESTIONS OR FAQS

Is Paget's Bone Disease Genetic?

Indeed, Paget's Disease of the Bone may run in families. It frequently runs in families, indicating that heredity may play a role in its development. Many genes that could be implicated have been found by researchers, the most well-studied of which is SQSTM1. The probability of contracting the illness may rise in response to mutations in this gene. A family history of Paget's Disease does not guarantee that an individual will get it, suggesting that environmental factors also come into play. It is advisable to discuss any close relatives who have been diagnosed with Paget's Disease with your healthcare professional. They may suggest genetic counseling or screening.

Exists A Cure For Paget's Disease?

Paget's Disease of the Bone cannot be cured at this time, however, it can be effectively controlled using medications that help manage symptoms and avoid consequences. Medications like bisphosphonates, which assist in controlling bone remodeling and lessen bone pain, are the mainstay of treatment.

Although it is used less frequently, calcitonin is an additional pharmaceutical alternative. Furthermore, supportive therapies such as analgesics, physical rehabilitation, and occasionally surgical procedures might aid in the management of symptoms. For the condition to be managed and quality of life to be increased, early identification and therapy are essential.

What Adjustments To Your Lifestyle Can Help Manage Paget's Disease?

Several lifestyle adjustments are frequently necessary to manage Paget's disease in order to reduce symptoms and enhance general health:

Healthy Diet: To maintain the health of your bones, make sure your diet is high in calcium and vitamin D. Good sources include foods like dairy, leafy greens, and fortified cereals.

Frequent Exercise: To preserve bone strength and general physical fitness, perform weight-bearing and muscle-strengthening exercises. Exercises like weight training, walking, and running can be helpful, but make sure to speak with your doctor to customize an activity plan for your health.

Steer Clear Of High-Impact Activities:

Steer clear of activities that place an undue amount of strain on your bones, like heavy lifting and high-impact sports, to prevent fractures and joint injury.

Sustaining a Healthy Weight: Maintaining a healthy weight is essential for controlling Paget's Disease because it lessens the strain on your bones and joints.

Frequent Medical Check-ups: Your healthcare practitioner can check you on a regular basis to assist you follow the disease's progression and make appropriate treatment adjustments.

Quitting Smoking and Reducing Alcohol: Smoking and binge drinking can both have detrimental effects on bone health. Your general bone health can be improved by lowering or getting rid of these.

Exist Any Other Options For Treating Paget's Disease?

While the mainstay of care for people with Paget's Disease is conventional medicine, some patients look into complementary therapies. To be sure these options are suitable and safe, talk with a healthcare professional:

Acupuncture: Although there is little scientific proof, some people get relief from bone pain with acupuncture.

Nutritional Supplements: In addition to calcium and vitamin D, supplements containing magnesium and omega-3 fatty acids may help maintain the general health of the bones. Always get medical advice before beginning a supplement regimen.

Herbal Remedies: Although the safety and effectiveness of some herbs are unknown, it is thought that they can promote bone health. It's crucial to use these under a healthcare provider's supervision.

Massage therapy: While it doesn't directly treat the illness, it helps relax stress in the muscles and enhance general comfort.

Mind-Body Methods: Exercises like yoga, tai chi, and meditation can reduce stress and enhance general well-being.

How Frequently Should I Contact My Healthcare Provider Again?

The severity of your illness, the therapies you are receiving, and the degree to which your symptoms are controlled will all influence how frequently you need follow-up appointments. Patients with Paget's Disease should typically visit their doctor once or twice a year. In addition to reviewing your treatment plan and keeping an eye on your symptoms, your provider may arrange imaging tests like bone scans or X-rays to track the progression of the condition. It could be necessary to schedule more regular visits if you encounter new issues or a flare-up of your symptoms. To guarantee the best possible management of the illness and to promptly modify your treatment plan, routine follow-up is crucial.

www.ingramcontent.com/pod-product-compliance
Lightning Source LLC
Chambersburg PA
CBHW071841210526
45479CB00001B/235